CW00517196

SONGS FOR MY UNBORN CHILDREN
BY
KATE BENTLEY

SONGS FOR MY UNBORN CHILDREN

For my children

SONGS FOR MY UNBORN CHILDREN

CONTENTS

SONGS FOR MY UNBORN CHILDREN

Foreword

Years ago, I was privileged to be given an early version of Songs for my Unborn Children from Kate during the course of her pregnancy, and to be allowed to use some for a book on Reproductive Ageing. She opened my eyes to the long, complex shadow that infertility, miscarriage and medicalised conception cast way beyond the immediate experiences. Doctors don't bring 'meaning' to our everyday routines that clash with each patient's exquisite vulnerability; it's not a strong part of our skill set. But Kate provides another route to compassionate understanding. Few artists can paint pain, but this poetess succinctly describes the emotional roller coaster of suffering, endurance and recovery that will resonate for women who've experienced it, and induce empathy from those who haven't. She gives voice to Everywoman's shame and taboos. Even though she was one of the lucky ones for whom IVF did work, for most it does not; for every million cute IVF babies celebrated in the news and advertisements there are another several millions of futile cycles, chemical pregnancies, miscarriages, wounded souls and emptier pockets. Although a proud mother now, Kate wears her scars. She doesn't gloat or forget her trauma, or the 'sisters in suffering' who follow her. They might, or might not, take a similar journey to eventual peace but will recognize themselves. Read, cry, learn, repeat.

Dr. Susan Bewley

SONGS FOR MY UNBORN CHILDREN

INFERTILITY

SONGS FOR MY UNBORN CHILDREN

Plan a family they said.

Except life doesn't always unfold
to the beat of a chosen rhythm.

A tug,
a gripe,
a taste,
a possible thought,
swollen
assumptions,
before
the blast.

Blue for success.
Red for desperation.
I try to hold on,
but it seeps out,
drop by bloody drop.

Always

There's a hole in my heart,
a raw, fist shaped wound
covered by a tissue layer of skin,
so my clothes won't chaff it,
or be permanently covered in blood.
But the wrong words pierce through
and it weeps,
and I weep,
so I have to be careful,
and avoid the words,
and the people who say them.

Swipe.
Pregnancy announcement.
Swipe.
Baby bump.
Swipe.
Trigger warning.
Triggered,
Wipe tears.
Swipe again.
Wipe
blood,
wipe tears.
Swipe.

Drinking coffee

Three cyclists,
all the gear,
no fear,
nineteen drivers,
eight women,
seven men,
four pram loads
and their pushers,
three nearly full buses,
two vicars,
deep in thought,
five pedestrians,
rushing,
four delivery men
two illegally parked,
three school girls,
in a huddle,
two teenagers,
smoking,
one common factor,
every person, everybody,
born from women.
Am I not a woman?

Spin a web of words,
sing a song,
paint, cut, paste, make,
yet I am the creative,
who cannot create creation.
How ironic.

What is an apricot
Without a stone?
An apple without its core?

I cried today.
I cried yesterday.
I will probably cry tomorrow.

Too happy,
too longed for,
too lucky,
too rich,
too poor,
too thin,
too fat,
too stretched,
too sclerotic,
too curdled,
too short sighted,
too acidic,
too committed,
too implausible,
too uncomfortable,
too controlling,
too relaxed,
too hot,
too cold,
too open,
too closed,
too red,
too pink,
too blue,
too desperate,
too stressed,
too scared,
too nervous,
too loaded,
too bloated,
too much.

Last night
I had a conversation
with my ovaries.
Right, what's up?
Anything I can do?
Left? Good to go this month?
What can I say to push the process?
Right, what are we going to do with Left
because this thing isn't happening?
I don't want to blame anyone,
but I'm tired of being left behind.
I want you both to know,
my sadness is eating me from the inside.
Left, do we have a problem with communication?
Right, back at you?
This needs to be an open platform,
please understand
we're in this together,
on the same side,
so just ignore my climate of fear.
But get it sorted, right?

Which one is me,
my mind or my body?
Which one is letting me down?
The negative thoughts that stalk my days,
or my confused chemistry
that no one seems to understand?
Maybe I should make the decision,
jump into a boxing ring,
beat this body into submission,
teach it a lesson it won't forget,
or do I just hurt myself?

Every Four Weeks,
that monthly reminder,
not only painful,
but painful.

How many infertile couples
does it take to screw in a lightbulb?

Screw in a lightbulb?
Would it help?

SONGS FOR MY UNBORN CHILDREN

I eat my feelings,
chocolate cake,
trifle, cream puffs,
candle lit dinners,
late nights,
raw liver,
chickens' feet,
I taste nothing.
I live my life;
exotic holidays,
a house,
weekends away,
a new car,
an empty cot.
I hear my desires,
Laughter,
giggles, gurgles,
a nursery rhyme,
crying,
there's nothing to touch.
I see time,
bare, blossom,
green, brown,
on a loop,
it doesn't change,
I smell promise,
a place, a doctor,
a date, a number.
I cradle hope,
I breathe desperation,
I birth tears.
I live.

On Saturday, I read in a newspaper:
'Seeing your child succeed is probably
the highest moment you can have.'
Let me think about that.

Life on hold,
the presence of absence
and old before my time,
I bob, untethered,
brushing milestones,
that aren't mine,
leaving no mark.

Emotions.
Better out than in,
but who to talk to
when fellow infertiles
are pretending too?

The anonymous woman
at dinner parties,
side-stepping the words,
their conclusions,
avoiding the pity and sympathy,
but out of the conversation,
a mere onlooker,
bandaged and bleeding.

Involuntary childlessness
is like walking around
with an invisible limb missing.

A summer cricket match,
Clear blue above,
The smell of cut grass,
men in white,
laughing and shouting,
the nostalgic sound of
leather on willow,
the chink of porcelain.
Three children run up to the boundary
all calling, 'Daddy, Daddy, Daddy',
every head turns, instinctively.
Except my husband's.

I hear
the sweet whisper
of my unborn children
in my heart and soul.
In my waking moments
and sleeping dreams
they come to me.

I am disappointment,
trading pain
with self-confidence,
my funds in the red.
My eyes are fear,
taunted each day
by what I can't have.
Their happiness
is sharp teeth,
large chunks of my flesh
hanging
from laughing mouths,
the trails of blood,
Raw spittle flecked spite,
are tears.
The only thing
I birth
is silent rage.
Still
I rampage,
unsnarling,
ungushing,
unhappy.

Celebrations

Mother's Day.
Flowers, cards, laughter
and a personal affront.
Christmas.
Presents, cards, laughter
and a personal affront.
My birthday.
Sadness,
as another year passes by.

I keep the world away,
a self-imposed exile from society,
because society rejects me.
My nose pressed against the glass,
I never escape.

Treat me
like you did
before I knew.

Step on the cracks.
Don't step on the cracks.
Get it right.
Late for a meeting;
doesn't care.
Smiled too much;
isn't serious.
Not nice enough;
lose points.
Too nice;
two steps back.
Catty remark;
slap her down.
Didn't laugh.
Points deducted.
Hole in tights.
Wrong shoes.
Burnt the cake.
Stained the shirt.
Dropped the load.
Unbalanced,
unordered,
undeserving.

A little girl smiled
at me today.
I smiled back,
shocked she could see me.

New skin,
under the skin,
onion skin,
peeled, unshelled, naked, raw,
skinned alive,
fur, snake, scales,
dry, wrinkled,
baby.

SONGS FOR MY UNBORN CHILDREN

There's a room up the stairs
down the corridor,
a church to the future,
with a touchable wooden cot
and foldable tiny clothes.
The altar, a changing table.
But not in our house.
We want to prove
our life is complete
until we have to make room.
Our talisman
are sanitary towels
and packets of tampax,
bought in bulk,
ready to wave
in the face of expectation.
Defensive, proactive,
inevitable.
Hateful.

Red eyes,
seeing red.

Such hope.
And then the rain
comes again.

The luxury of carelessness
chased away by dead leaves and unwanted rubbish.

Not happening.
Not working.
Not enough.
Knotted.
Noted.
Naked.
Nothing.

Make love.
Make a baby.
It's a fine line.

I am angry,
I am frustrated,
I cry,
I am frustrated with the world,
but most of all,
I am frustrated with myself.

Although doctors frustrate me
a great deal.

It takes two

I am the long grass bending in the wind,
caught by every emotion.
He is my rock,
calm, dependable, there.
I am the driving force,
pushing forward, no matter what,
for a dream
I refuse to relinquish.
If I said stop, he would stop,
and still be happy,
still be happy with barren me.
If I say more,
he says, OK. Are you sure?
And has to watch as I get buffeted by the gales,
holding tightly to my roots.

Different eyes

You see a broader picture,
we see the abyss.
You see our future,
we see a lonely path,
one step in front of another.
You see us surrounded by our children,
we see ourselves guarding the flames of hope
with bare hands and empty arms.
You see solutions,
we see doctors.
You see us drained and low,
we see the strength in our marriage.
You see us as a couple.
We see ourselves as a family already.

Sunny side up,
over easy,
soft boiled,
scrambled,
but best of all,
fertilised.

My heart sighs
when?
The reply comes,
tomorrow.

In my head
I know I am not to blame.
In my heart,
I don't know who else there is.

I have no control
over this basic function
of my body,
so I control
vitamins,
weight,
alcohol consumption,
acupuncture,
reflexology,
and Chinese herbs instead.
So now I can't even drown my sorrows,
and when I don't drink,
people think I am pregnant.
Great.

Do you smoke?
Give up smoking,
take control.
Do you drink?
Give up drinking,
take control.
Overweight?
Give up eating,
Take control.
Depressed?
I'm not surprised.

Darwin and his gene pool suck.
All I can hope
is that evolution takes control,
and men start having babies too,
which will not only benefit infertile women,
but also the workplace, society
and the world in general.

Relax,
they say.
Don't stress,
they insist.
Easy words,
I think.
Open your eyes
and sit where I am sitting,
read a book,
watch TV,
go to the cinema,
visit friends,
a trip to the theatre,
music, opera,
advertising,
radio,
newspapers,
magazines.
Only one word
makes the world go around:
Procreation.

Stereotypes

I am not a mother,
but nor am I
a career woman
or over forty.
But if I was,
should I be judged
for using my brain, my talents
and forging a successful career?
Should I be criticized
for finding unsuccessful relationships
and not for finding Mr. Right?
After all, it takes two
to make a baby and create a family,
and some people genuinely believe
that stability and life experiences
are defining factors in bringing up children.
Contrary to popular opinion,
not all woman consciously think
I'll be OK, no matter what,
let me choose where the kids will fit in,
there's always the easy option of
fertility treatment and IVF
with their gilt-edged guarantees.
I can always buy
an egg, sperm, an embryo, a baby.
No. It is not thoughtlessness that delays
the decision to have a family,
far from it,
for the majority, it is life.

SONGS FOR MY UNBORN CHILDREN

The words I don't want to hear

'What do you do and do you have children?'
I fail on both counts,
I spend my life trying for the latter.

'So when are you going to have children?'
When the slow wind blows?
And if I knew the answer, would I tell you?

'Do you want children?'
Do I lie, or open the floodgates?
If I unburden, will you expect me
then to comfort you?
Instead I talk about an indulgent holiday we're planning,
the thing we can control.

'You're not getting any younger'
I live my life in two week slots,
counting the wrinkles on my ovaries,
knowing with every second of each day that
the passing of time
will lead me to a future,
whether I want it or not,
are the words I don't say,
rather I smile,
and ask about your new shoes.

'I just had to look at my husband and I was pregnant'
So that's what we're doing wrong,
so simple, and the doctors never mention it.

'Then I popped them out, like shelling peas'
Do you expect me to laugh?
Except the worst thing is, I do.

'I am pregnant. Again.
An accident. I'm devastated'
What do you want me to say?
so am I?
I covet the things you take for granted,
when you choose names,
I choose fertility clinics,
I jump through hoops of fire,
you shell peas.
'And your loss,
I'm so sorry,
but at least it wasn't a baby yet'
If it wasn't a baby,
what was I carrying?
And why are my clothes
now heavy with tears?
'At least it was an early loss'
Tell me,
is there a hierarchy of pain?
a competition with gold medals and world records,
a sliding scale of sympathy?
But I say nothing,
watching your words
twist, growing scales,
crawling, dark, fat and fleshy,
whilst I shrink.
'It's so common,
there must've been something wrong'
Well then it must be ok,
how silly of me for feeling like this,
I smile, as I disappear,
into the ground,
holed in my hole.

'I envy your life-style'
Do you?
I experience prejudice everyday
because society is formed around the family unit,
from rail tickets Christmas,
the family is celebrated.
'I know someone who went through six IVF
cycles,
all failed, then they went on holiday
and came back pregnant'
So that's all I need to do.
'After her ninth cycle, she had twins'
Does this give me hope?
or dishearten me?
Why this need
to impose something of your own story
upon mine?
Except I nod,
and ask, 'Which clinic?'
'Try not to think about it'
About what? The baby-pink elephant in the corner?
'We know this fabulous nutritionist'
Yet another person to fleece me,
as I take the number.
'You'll get pregnant when you give up trying'
So you know how to laugh in the face of fate then?
'You're too busy'
I'm trying not to think about it.
'You're not busy enough'
How do you give up the future in your mind?
What do you do instead?
How do you rewrite your plans

and find peace
so that life's daily rituals
don't become a barb every time?
How do you grieve a fantasy?
'I have something to tell you
which is quite hard for me,
as I don't want to hurt you,
I'm six months pregnant'
Why is it so hard to tell me?
Give me more credit than to act
like a wailing banshee in public,
it would have been equally as hard five months ago,
but at least I would have respected you more.
This just confirms my alienation and isolation.
But I jump up and congratulate you,
flinging my arms around your neck,
telling you how special this is.
'It's obviously not the right time for you,
if it's meant to be, it's meant to be'
So you say.
But I'm not getting any younger,
so what should I do?

SONGS FOR MY UNBORN CHILDREN

Do I hear the words they say?

Are they spoken with ignorance
or am I guilty of not listening properly?
Are they delivered with innocence
and no intention to hurt?
A lack of realisation of what is being said,
and everything implied to the negative
in my mind only?
Am I possessed by a resistance
I otherwise purport to condemn,
the only sin, trying too hard?
I know I pull away from people who don't understand,
and gravitate towards those that do,
a typically self-destructive reaction
when I, the victim, assume a one-sided view.
I also know, as I become more vulnerable,
as my sense of heightened awareness grows,
I become less able to cope.
then, through this low-resolution murkiness,
you think you can imagine what it's like,
you want to be able to explain everything
or tell me why this is so,
and sometimes you don't realise
the impact of the things you say,
a blind witness to the carnage
of a few misdirected words.
The truth is, I feel weighed down,
protecting you from disappointing me,
always catching the back-draft of emotions,
I can't carry you as well
or add yet another layer
to this thick, suffocating shame,
so I remain grimly silent,
accepting I cannot make you behave

in the ways I would like,
knowing that the only person
I have the power to change
is myself.
But even when I recognize my own insecurities
I can only respond
when I have the strength to do so.
Until then, nature will take the lead
and the storms must steer their course,
and sometimes actions speak louder than words,
and sometimes the unsaid is more eloquent.

Let me explain

When I am having invasive tests,
I am riding a rollercoaster of emotions.
When I am taking hormones,
I am riding a rollercoaster of emotions.
When I see a pregnant woman, ripe with hope,
I am riding a rollercoaster of emotions.
When I see a baby, mewly new,
I am riding a rollercoaster of emotions.
When I see a beautiful child, the future present,
I am riding a rollercoaster of emotions,
When I am at family gatherings,
I am riding a rollercoaster of emotions.
Sometimes, when I am having a cup of tea,
I am riding a rollercoaster of emotions.

If you want to help,
don't pretend to know,
and don't make assumptions,
listen and learn,
tell me
how unfair this is,
tell me
we will make
fantastic parents,
tell me
I will be a lovely mum,
tell me
if anyone can get through this
I can.
I don't admire much
at the moment,
so tell me
you admire me,
and maybe
I will too.

Their babies, my babies

How do I tell you,
your babies are not my babies.
Your pregnancy
is not my pregnancy.
My grief
is not at your joy,
it is the reminder of my loss.
So let me be happy for you,
allow me that grace,
that normality.
Then let me mourn
what might have been.

SONGS FOR MY UNBORN CHILDREN

The advantages of pretending

Shoulders back and a smile on my face,
it's good to swim with the current,
because sometimes exposure solves nothing.
This is my private property
and I can decide
to lock away my sadness
for my own protection.
I can avoid the worry
that some understand less
as time goes on,
and grasp rare moments of freedom.
Even when my mouth stretches open
in a silent scream
no-one knows how deep the cut goes,
I just pull my soot clad cloak tighter,
fashion designed
to cover up my thoughts and faults,
and remain one of the crowd.

I cover my shame by living a lie,
I laugh to cover the tears,
my fears decorated
by smiles, bright eyes,
and designer trappings.
Distracting distractions.
The more I glitter,
the greater I hurt.

Safety in secrets

Why avoid the pity and sympathy,
Aren't they the antidote to hurt and pain?
It's all we know,
without these,
we don't know how to cope.
Nor do we,
but will you catch me when I fall?

Do I want you to see my hurt?
Not if it becomes an object of general discussion,
not if it becomes trivialised with everyone owning a
piece,
not if it feeds the monkey on my back,
turning it into a pampered pet.
Do I want you to see how this has chipped away at me,
or do I want you to see the me I want to feel?
Walk in my shoes then tell me.

I know you want to understand,
but how can you know the wound
from the wounded?

How can you know how hard
it is to pretend on a daily basis,
around the people
that you love?

Can you understand?
I know that you try,
but the truth is you can't.
and that hurts me as well.

Waiting,
always waiting,
and not moving
never gets me closer.

Sometimes up,
sometimes down,
sometimes I can cope,
sometimes I can't.
But always,
I pick myself up,
I hope.

The chasm

Hold a friend's hand,
recognise their pain,
lead them to the bridge
and watch them cross to the other side.

I am strong.
I am intelligent.
I know my mind.
But my body is useless,
my body is me,
therefore I am useless.

What is said,
what is meant,
including a world of inarticulate fear,
I am told one thing,
something else happens,
and no one can say yes for sure.

Fertility
is not the be all
and end all.
But it feels like it.
It is all consuming,
and I am obsessed
by its unfairness.
If I stand back,
I accept it will not
define my existence.
But I know
it will impact all my life.

The lottery of life,
that randomly points a bony finger
and says
who can have children,
and who can't.

Take your money,
fame, celebrity and fortune,
I just want to be normal,
I just want to be a mother.

When I leave my fertile years behind me
will I finally be able to let it all go?
Or will the next generation
appear to haunt me still?

I know
the capacity to love,
does not depend
on sharing my genes.
But I don't want to prove it.

SONGS FOR MY UNBORN CHILDREN

MISCARRIAGE
AND
IVF FAILURE

SONGS FOR MY UNBORN CHILDREN

I mother
blood and grief.

SONGS FOR MY UNBORN CHILDREN

Everything goes to shit.
The ball crusher
swings,
a bullseye blow,
body curving
to impact point,
hip bone in socket,
shattered,
air forced out.
feet off the ground,
bone splintering,
paring,
collapsing,
in numb shock,
I free fall.

Down the pan,
blood, discharge, cells, mucus,
congratulations,
maternity clothes,
scan pictures,
dreams.
A puddle of piss and bits,
gush, furl, hurl, plunge,
rejected, ejected.

Still, I search among the debris.
But nothing is salvageable.

No one to help,
doctors useless,
what you see on TV,
a fairytale.

SONGS FOR MY UNBORN CHILDREN

Anger

I feel it within,
let it slowly grow,
taking shape,
giving it life,
till out through my lips,
the rage spews out.

Born, perfectly formed,
rabid and ready to multiply,
bled, spilled, stained,
contagion spread
and carried forward.

I projectile vomit the noise,
bouncing it off my home-made walls,
picking it up with sweaty hands
and slamming it back again.
Crushed, mangled,
crouched whilst it's crunched,
I wring the syllables from my neck,
words no one knows,
But all understand,
spitting out,
hocked up balls of phlegm
mixed with sinuous snot.
Grief and anger, the uncontainable escaping,
more tears and mess over the irony.

Ripe fruit
inside rotten.
A great looking great product,
modern marketing at its best.
Image rich,
truth poor,
walking, talking
fake news.
I was fooled too.

A rosebud,
coloured baby pink,
dipped in green,
kissed with dew.
I smash it
with a hammer,
smashing,
I smile.

Slack jaw,
clotted, stilted thoughts.
A bruised silence,
a bleeding void.

The nights are the worst
when the core I hold to myself
so tightly during the day,
dissolves into the dark
as all my boundaries expand out
till I am a mere speck of dust
fighting on a sea of anguish.

Our bond of blood,
we are rejected together,
you from me,
me from you,
but please know,
it was manslaughter,
not murder.

You will not know
how much I loved you.
But I did.

Despised and rejected.
A woman of sadness,
acquainted with tears,
borne the grief,
carried the sorrows,
wounded and bruised,
scorned.
This rebuke has broken
my heart,
so full of heaviness,
is there any sorrow
like this sorrow?

How to explain
the loss of a child
one has neither seen
nor touched.
I held them in me,
I hold them in my heart.
Now cheated,
angry at me,
angry at them.
How to explain
the love and the longing
already in place,
the future planned,
our shadow child
at our side.
How to explain
that this has happened,
and yet so few
will talk about it,
let alone remember.

A hole,
smaller than a pinprick
sucks all the light in.

Ovaries that rust,
the tide lines left
like the rings in a tree.

A womb that leaks,
dribbles over everything,
smearing acidic destruction.

Where on a scale of one to ten is your pain?
And I think,
what is your reference point?
Because you are not me.
This thing I hold is mine alone.
My amputation, if that's what I had,
would be unimaginable to you.
Pain is not shareable,
so I communicate in vain.

SONGS FOR MY UNBORN CHILDREN

Was there something I should have done but didn't do?
Was there something I didn't do but should have done?
And then I think,
famine, flood, war and strife,
and women still have children.
So why couldn't I have mine?

'We don't want to mention it,
In case we remind you'.
As if I could forget.
And then I think,
famine, flood, war and strife,
and women still have children.
So why couldn't I have mine?

'At least you can get pregnant'.
So they say.
And then I think,
famine, flood, war and strife,
and women still have children.
So why couldn't I have mine?

Heroin addicts and alcoholics
have families,
children in care
were all born.
And then I think,
famine, flood, war and strife,
and women still have children.
So why couldn't I have mine?

SONGS FOR MY UNBORN CHILDREN

It is a fearful thing
to love
what can be lost.

I lost them,
but I carry them still
in my heart.
I see them,
but only in my mind.
And as each year passes,
I lose them more,
a loss that time can't heal
but rather grows in its enormity,
as I lose my youth as well.

My advice

1. Don't tell people your secrets
2.

I thieve the feelings,
loot the memories,
hide them away,
my only treasures.

I know
I bruise more easily now.

Unlisted, listing
detached person,
currently in a derelict state.
Sits in beautiful situation
with no close neighbours
and uninterrupted views
across the valley.
Garden well maintained
with mature specimens,
subject to flooding.
Wiring and plumbing
requires complete overhaul,
and due to recent storms,
a structural report
is also strongly recommended.
There is existing planning permission
for an extension,
which will lapse shortly.
Although at first stage fix,
this person remains incomplete,
but offers substantial family accommodation
with generous open plan areas
for those with vision, money and time.

Starting again

My mind is in neutral,
attempting to be carefree
but careworn,
seen rather than seeing,
unhappy-go-unlucky,
forced to wear
my heart on my sleeve,
and still waiting.

I want to choose my own story,
to find a handhold before the fall,
a glass knocked
onto a stone floor
caught midair.
Turbulence on a plane
that scares,
then settles.
Except I slip,
tumble headlong,
glancing blows,
cracking bones,
knocked, winded,
damaged,
broken.

If I keep them in
Do my fears turn to strength?
or does my strength
run like sand between my fingers?
If I let the pain
fall from my shoulders,
does it dissolve into the ground?
or puddle at my feet
till I drown in my tears?
If I pretend,
does the pretence become real?
Or is it an impenetrable barrier,
a mask to be worn, unmoving?
And then the knife of failure twists again.
It breaks my heart,
but I've learnt I won't die,
yet it kills me each time.
Dust to dust, ashes to ashes
If I hurt enough,
will the rewards ever be mine?
Or do I stand, sentinel,
and watch the winds of time
pass me by?

I stand up to be counted,
walk up to the line,
will myself to believe,
then take the body blow.
So I stand up to be counted,
walk up to the line,
will myself to believe,
then take the body blow.
So I stand up to be counted,
walk up to the line,
will myself to believe,
then take the body blow.
So I stand up to be counted,
walk up to the line,
will myself to believe,
then take the body blow.

Einstein said,
the definition of insanity
is doing the same thing
over and over again.
and expecting
different results.

He was right.

A matter of percentages,
and as they reduce,
I still cling to hope.
And stand up to be counted.

Adoption?

There are other paths.

Nature or nurture?
This much I know,
children can have their
hearts broken too.

TREATMENT

SONGS FOR MY UNBORN CHILDREN

I will become a mother
at any cost,
but there will come a time,
when we have to draw
the line.

Courage is not
the absence of fear,
but rather
the ability to act
in the face of it.

Treatment:
Let's throw in
the postcode lottery as well.
Outrage it's a gamble.
Relief the dice fall in our favour.

The cycling is not easy,
but it's not the pain,
or the money,
it's the lack of a guarantee.

They say,
infertility is as stressful
as cancer.
How many people know that?

Hormones up,
should be down.
Costs up.
Thumbs up,
money down
Hopes up.
Pants down.
Wand up.
Drugged up.
Drown.

Doctors

I asked the doctor,
Is there absolutely anything
I can do
to increase my chances?
My health?
She said no.

Just another infertile couple,
just another train wreck.

Doctors wear white coats
and tick boxes.
Sufferers read books,
search the net,
change their diet,
pop vitamin pills
visit acupuncturists,
nutritionists, herbalists,
aromatherapists and
offer themselves up for hypnotism,
who is right?
The person who gets the result?

Why don't they realise,
that anything
I can do
is something?

SONGS FOR MY UNBORN CHILDREN

Fold over, score.
Unfold,
Fold top and bottom to the centre.
Score.
Fold in half,
then half again.
Crease.
Rotate upside down.
Fold both sides to the centre.
Fold all corners down.
Open up.
Score.
Press on the diagonal lines.
Fold outer flaps toward the centre.
flatten.
Open each corner.
flatten.
Turn inside out,
then upside down.
Score.
Fold out.
Turn over.
Score.
Fold the edges.
Turn over.
Reverse fold.
Refold.
Score.
Repeat.
Fold.
Fold again, fold again.
Flatten, pull out.
Repeat, pull out.
Repeat.
Fold.

Called in to see the doctor,
lie on the couch,
legs akimbo.
Return to wait in the waiting room,
aptly named,
see the doctor again,
'Have I been in to see him?'
He doesn't recognise my face.
'Hamster in a wheel', I think,
and climb aboard the
medical conveyor belt again.

That lay people
do not understand
is hard enough.
But I expected more
from doctors.
Instead,
tact and empathy
are lost to fact and statistics,
the emotional strain
ignored.

They dehumanize themselves,
they dehumanize their patients.

What price a curtain?

They see
a problem to be solved,
and a slab of meat
to be prodded and poked,
No wonder
I wonder
what I have become.

This is so personal,
to me,
my life,
my bits,
but let's pretend it's not.

Waiting rooms.
Short on chairs,
strong on mayhem.

Waiting rooms.
High on waiting,
low on magazines.

Waiting rooms.
So much emotion,
so little noise.

Happiness and positivity
create good hormones.
So what happens
if you get into a rut
because you are trying
to be positive?

How do you stay positive
when the expectation
has always failed?

I have found
a place of peace,
an acknowledgement
that although
I cannot change the future,
I can change
the way I deal with it.

There is only one way:
to be positive,
because whether I am positive
or not,
the depth of the disappointment
remains the same.

To fail is to fall
to succeed is to fly.
I have to believe
I have wings
Otherwise, why try?

SONGS FOR MY UNBORN CHILDREN

The Long Road

The first step: a trip to the doctors,
means on the one hand,
something is wrong,
on the other, the chance of a solution.
The questions the trip raises,
breeds a series of tests,
and so the journey starts,
each one offering an answer,
or the uncertainty of some dreadful disease,
HIV, Syphilis, Chlamydia or cancer.
Girding one's loins, literally,
to go through with it.
And waiting, always waiting.
waiting for results, waiting for a way forward,
waiting for a miracle.
The offer of less invasive treatment
gratefully grasped.
Holding new drugs with new hope,
only to drink from the cup of disappointment again,
and again, and again.
Reaching the last station on the line,
a new cross roads: face the last bastion,
the holy grail of infertility: IVF
or accept the death of the dream
of our own biological child.
We stand up to be counted.

It Starts

The first challenge, a simple blood test.
Get a score of ten or under to pass Go
and collect £200,
over ten, the mirror of truth is held up,
no matter how young you may look or feel
on the outside,
there is no escape from your biological age
on the inside,
over ten and the spectre of the menopause
raises its head,
over ten and the hands of time quicken,
chances lessen
as the amount of drugs needed
now rises,
along with your heart rate
and the cost,
The goal posts moved
another ten feet back.

Going down the down-regging route

Options discussed, decisions made, protocols decided
start the drugs.
Instead of facing the prospect
of an unpredicted menopause,
the aim is to bring it on, glimpse the future,
HRT an option in the years ahead?
Your partner may think so.
what fertility you had previously
so preciously held,
is swept away by injections,
that are actually worse in thought than deed,
but strength of mind is needed
because it is just such an alien action,
do you get used to it?
No, it's just something that has to be done.
How long is this stage?
It depends. Sometimes two weeks,
sometimes more.
You just do it,
at least you are doing something.

The next step: Has your system shut down?

What a thought.
If it has move forward,
if it hasn't, keep taking the drugs,
and hope for the best,
maybe the cycle will end here,
before it has even started,
the level of suffering
irrelevant to the outcome,
there are no guarantees.
If it has, the time has come to swing the other way,
from zero to hero to grow eggs
like a battery hen,
yet there is a strange pleasure,
apart from the raging hormones,
and the additional injections,
that at last,
you've reached a positive stage,
a creative stage,
you are growing your family,
even if it is under hothouse conditions.
How long is this stage?
Sometimes two weeks,
sometimes more.
And always questions:
Are the drugs working?
How many follicles have you produced?
Too few? Too many?
What is their quality?
And will your lining be thick enough?
Or is there something else that will let you down?

SONGS FOR MY UNBORN CHILDREN

It goes wrong

I didn't respond to the drugs,
I fell like a stone from Everest,
only two follicles,
and one large, that wouldn't last,
the other small.
'I'm sorry' said the doctor,
so was I.
The journey ended,
the journey home a blur
of tears and failure,
again.
Even with a blasting of drugs
and medical missiles,
my body could still let me down,
The loneliness, the emptiness.
The realisation of the end of the line.
Later that same afternoon,
John takes the call from the hospital,
he has left work to be with me,
the despair in my voice
echoing down the telephone line,
drawing him to me,
a time of pure need
and he is there,
without me ever asking.
A tweak of fate,
'They want you to continue with the drugs'
'Why?'
'Because your blood test,
has shown there may be more there',
'Is it true,
or are they just prolonging the agony?'
A question neither of us

can answer.
We feel like the victims of a car crash,
emotionally battered,
unable to see any positives any longer,
always expecting the worst.

SONGS FOR MY UNBORN CHILDREN

The next scan

He comes with me for the scan on Monday,
holds my hand.
The news is not brilliant,
but better.
We have four tiny ones.
Egg collection is set up for Wednesday,
then extended to Friday,
and, somehow, we get there.
Egg Collection.

Egg collection is brutal,
conscious yet not conscious,
aware yet not aware,
aware of the indignities,
not aware of the pain,
until later.
They collect four,
Four eggs of hope.
How many will fertilise?
How many will be our family?
We won't know.
The hospital will only call with bad news,
the telephone is now the enemy.
Embryo transfer will be Monday,
only the weekend to recover,
it seems unbelievable that
such a precious cargo could be
returned so soon
when my insides
feel like a war zone.
We get through the weekend,
thinking and hoping
for our tiny family,

our children,
struggling for life.
On Monday, the telephone rings
I leap out of bed,
and throw my mobile at John,
'It's the hospital,
with bad news,
they'll try this phone next',
he looks at me bleary and bemused,
'There's no way it's the hospital',
he says,
'This is the NHS and
it's three in the morning,
You've been dreaming',
And I had.
We return to the hospital
and with almost something like hope,
against the odds,
all have survived.
We have four embryos,
four little children,
a family,
Two for the freezer,
and two for me.

Transfer

The transfer is done
on a full bladder.
Need I say more.
Above me on the ceiling,
a picture of an island,
somewhere in the Pacific,
palm trees and turquoise seas.
Given the choice,
I know where I'd prefer to be,
exactly where I am.
The Transfer is completed at 11.32 precisely.
And now they are mine,
all mine.
For this moment,
it is as if a great weight
has been lifted from my shoulders.
Now I am on familiar ground,
the two week wait holds no fear for me.
The test at the end does.
But till then,
I will enjoy, nurture and hope.

AFTERWARDS

SONGS FOR MY UNBORN CHILDREN

The two week wait

Pregnant until proven otherwise,
and yet, the exultation of my first pregnancy
is like a groping memory,
a joy briefly glanced,
then snatched away.
As was the second,
and the third,
and those in-between.
Don't blame yourself, they say,
who else can I blame
for a loss so personal?
They were mine, I lost them.
I lie here now,
and look back on the road taken,
I lie here now,
and think how long that road has been,
I lie here now,
and remember each painful step,
I lie here now,
and know if you are with me,
all that time will be gone
in the blink of my water-filled eye.

I chase
single magpies
out of the garden.

The Test

I have to go to the hospital today
for my pregnancy test,
then head home
and wait again for the result.
Just to get to this stage is something,
but I am fearful to go any further.
I have reached the point
of extreme emotion.
Joy and amazement,
or,
despite everything,
on top of everything,
darkness and despair.
A knife edge of pain or pleasure.
I cannot take the call,
good news or bad,
the doctors will have to phone John,
only he can tell me.

John has spoken to them.
Time stood still.
And then he said those magic words,
and then he said them again,
because I didn't believe him the first time.

SONGS FOR MY UNBORN CHILDREN

PREGNANCY

I have crossed over

I am standing on the other side,
and the ground feels strange beneath my feet.
Behind me,
pale faces and desperate eyes,
beside me,
so much
celebration and delight
I can hardly relate.
Frighteningly grateful to be here,
tears of joy,
cries of laughter,
yet so fearful of the future.
I have been here before,
only to cross back,
and I cannot cross again.

Week four:

My baby is an embryo,
each cell dividing daily,
again and again.
A mere 1 mm in length,
her presence already recognised
in my bladder and breasts.
I am pro-choice,
but I still love my children
when they are cells.

Her?
How could I know?
I don't.
But I do.

SONGS FOR MY UNBORN CHILDREN

First early scan

I am pregnant.
So grateful for the chance,
so scared of the otherwise,
haunted by the memories of before,
each scan
a reminder
of the scans of the past.
That lurch, like a heartbeat
except there is no heartbeat.
The realisation. the numbness, the floating
like you floating,
the suspension,
the suspension of time,
holding through, and then the release,
a silent projection of wracking sorrow.
This first scan: The very moment to see our child,
to prove you are really here,
to grasp the truth and joy,
or, the time to fall off
the mountain of expectation,
so patiently climbed,
into darkness and despair.
Game over.

I close my eyes,
unable to look,
for once, willing to wait,
my heart beating.

Then your heart beating.

A miracle.

SONGS FOR MY UNBORN CHILDREN

We have seen you

You are with us,
my precious baby,
we have seen your growing heart
and heard it's living beat.
And in my joy, I panic still,
to see you, feel you, hear you and lose you,
would break my soul.
Nothing can change this except time,
so I count each second,
and as each day crawls by,
my hope and love for you grows,
and as it grows,
so does the enormity of losing you.
Already you are so much a part of me
that each paranoia of mine,
each twinge or pain or superstition,
reflects on you and I fear again,
But I have to remember,
and hold onto the thought,
as I hold onto you,
that as small as you are,
you are already your own person,
you have your own will, your own drive
you are not me, just a part of me,
independent and individual.
striving for life, a personality,
a tiny human being in your own right.
so grow strong, be special,
I will wait for you.
And do my best
not to kill you.

If I could give
a year of my life,
to get to twelve weeks now,
successfully,
this day, this minute,
I would do it willingly.

Week seven:
More like a coffee bean,
but looking like a tadpole,
with a head and a trunk,
for which I apologise.

Week eight:
You change from embryo to foetus,
and your umbilical cord is developing.
A crucial time for me
in terms of losing you.
And you have started to move,
little reflex movements.

Week nine:
The size of a grape
with eyelids,
though your eyes are tightly closed.

I have never known
time to move so slowly.

Each day

I am meant to be
sorting out our building works,
to get the house ready for you, my baby,
yet I am finding it so hard.
Is it exhaustion: emotional and mental?
Or is it simpler than that.
Am I so used to living day by day,
that I struggle to contemplate
anything in the future?

Week ten:
Your arms and legs are waving,
as are your tiny hands, feet, fingers and toes,
you can breathe a sigh of relief
as your tail disappears this week.
I can breathe a sigh of relief
as your umbilical cord
starts taking over from me,
surely more reliable.
It is possible to hear your heartbeat,
and I did.
Like the hooves of a running horse.

SONGS FOR MY UNBORN CHILDREN

Twelve week scan

Why am I so scared?
In my heart,
I know I will see your
beating heart again,
even if my brain tells me otherwise.
I just hope, with all my strength,
It will be in a strong, healthy body.
The innocent joy of happy expectation
is now lost and gone forever,
and in its stead,
I still fear and expect the worst,
with trauma at every turn.
They say the brave have
too little imagination,
I know I have too much.
I feel as if you are already sitting an exam,
one that I am desperate for you to pass,
with no chance for revision,
and the burden of my bad luck
on your shoulders.
But would a bad outcome make any difference?
Only because I want to protect you
and want the best for you,
Because I made you and willed you into being.
Who are they to say whether my baby is perfect or not?
And yet I still want you to be as perfect to the world
as you will always be to me.

Joy

I am walking around with
two hearts,
two brains
two mouths,
two noses,
four ears,
four eyes,
twenty fingers,
twenty toes,
and feel on top of the world.

Which one are you?

Girl or boy,
I don't really care,
as long as you are mine.
But I tell everyone,
as I stroke my tummy,
you are a fertility doctor,
with a heart.

Week fourteen:
You have tiny soft nails
and may even suck your thumb.
I think I can feel you,
but it could be wishful thinking.

Week sixteen:
I am sure I can feel you,
within me,
you are emptying your bladder
every 40-45 minutes.
Charming.

Week nineteen:
Some people say you can dream.

Week twenty:
Your ears are functional.
Do you know what you hear?
Mainly my heart.

SONGS FOR MY UNBORN CHILDREN

Twenty week anomaly scan

It has happened.
The nightmare scan.
and now I can barely stand
let alone function.

It started so well.
I could feel you
and knew we would see a heartbeat.
I was happy,
finally confident
and looking forward to seeing you again.
There were two sonographers,
a trainee and her superior,
we chatted as your blurry form appeared,
my beautiful child before me.
I explained,
as she set to work,
the six long years,
the eight miscarriages,
the IVF,
how special you were,
how lucky I was.
She smiled,
'All is OK',
and I smiled back.
'I just want to take a look',
said Mrs Senior.
So I lay back again,
happy with the silence,
trying to interpret the moving mists myself.
'There's calcium in the heart,
it's nothing to worry about per se,
but there's also dilatation around the kidneys as well,

SONGS FOR MY UNBORN CHILDREN

and I'm concerned femur length is small,
These are nothing to worry about just yet per se,
but added together,
these three things,
could be a marker for Downs.
You'll need to see a Consultant'.
Ok, I say,
how can I speak?
You say these things,
but you haven't said
there's anything wrong per se,
and I am flying to Greece for a holiday
in two days time.
We can't get you an appointment before then.
Ok,
it can't be that serious then,
I'll see them when I get back.
We need this holiday,
as I said before,
we've been through quite a lot just recently.
She turned,
looked me straight in the eye and said:

But what about an amnio?
What about termination?

And then,
at that moment,
I knew
whatever we are in life:
infertile miscarriage sufferer,
IVF survivor,
daughter,
sister,

wife,
mother,
child,
we are nothing on that couch.

And the bottom fell out of my world.

We are in limbo.

We don't know what this means,
we have nothing to cling onto,
we don't even know what my odds are,
for something serious to be wrong.
They want me to have an amnio?
But I have a history of miscarriage.

All I do know is
I can't eat,
I can't sleep,
I can't stop crying,
I can't stop this pregnancy
and I don't know what to do.

I look back to my fears at my twelve week scan,
and feel sick.
I was ready then,
now, I am not.

SONGS FOR MY UNBORN CHILDREN

One in three hundred risk of miscarriage.
Does it matter?

We can't lose this baby.
This baby moves.
This baby moves me.
This baby is our child,
so longed for,
dreamt of.

If the news is bad,
we won't terminate,
so why risk the procedure?

How strong do we need to be?

Flights are cancelled,
appointments are made,
a second opinion sought.
and only the best will do,
our one concern
the emotional cost.
Yes, there is calcium in the heart,
yes, there is dilatation of the kidneys,
the femurs are small,
and did you know
there is a notch on your placenta too?
But overall,
your baby is fine,
your odds are halved from your twelve weeks scan,
which translates as
one in four hundred.
It's your call.

We come out walking on air.

One in four hundred?

You wouldn't bet on it.
Would you?
Not unless it was the lottery.

No-one
can take this pregnancy
away from me.
I will live and love
Every curve
and every bump.

Week twenty two:
Loud noises can wake you up.
So far I have
resisted playing you Mozart.

Week twenty four:
We celebrate parent's day.
Whatever happens now,
we both have identities.

Because of the notch and the dilatation on the kidneys,
I am receiving monthly scans.
And my fear of scans,
is turning into a phobia.
Every time they come,
not only do I have to go,
but each time they ask me
'Did you have the amnio?'
And raise the spectres once again.

There is nothing they can do
until the birth.
There is something I can do.

I refuse anymore scans.

Week twenty eight:
Your eyes are open,
the windows to your soul.
I would love you to have your father's eyes.
And you can perceive light.
Forget the dark.

Week thirty:
You can recognise my voice
and you sleep when I wake,
my movements rocking you,
then you wake when I try to sleep,
your kicking pounding my innards.
Can you hear me telling you to sleep?
If we could sort this one now,
it would make both our lives
so much easier in the long run.

Week thirty one:
Your skin is now new-born pink.
My new favourite colour.

SONGS FOR MY UNBORN CHILDREN

Your Photos

My photos follow your story
from your abstract start,
a mere eight cells,
to a picture of an actual baby.
An uncanny case,
of art imitating life,
loved, coveted, looked at
and adored.

Week thirty two:
We are waiting for my belly button to pop.

Week thirty six:
I just walk out
and I am an event,
smiles surround me.

Week thirty seven:
You could be gaining as much as
one full ounce per day.
I certainly am.

Week thirty eight:
It's a waiting game.

SONGS FOR MY UNBORN CHILDREN

How small your baby-gro's,
how dear your socks?

Today
I bought a packet of
nappies for newborns,
and almost peed
myself with pleasure.

I also bought
maternity pants,
nipple cream
maternity and breast pads
and a breast pump.
They have a strange, mystical quality about them.

The high,
of standing in a
baby shop,
choosing your cot.
Far better than any known drug.

These memories I will treasure
forever.

Week thirty nine:
We are ready.
The Hospital bag is packed.

Week forty:
Where are you?
Apart from the obvious.

She is here.

We are a family of three.
So blissfully happy
and in raptures
over our beautiful
Wee redheaded girl.

And she is perfect
in every which way.
She nestles in my arms,
and fits under my chin.

Isabella,
Born 19 October
At 3.59 am precisely
Weighing 6 lbs. 8 oz.

In her honour,
please raise a glass or two
in celebration of the miracle
that is new life,
and in particular,
the true wonder that is finally
our beloved daughter.

At the start of the day,
and the setting of the sun,
this is life.

love
Mumma x

SONGS FOR MY UNBORN CHILDREN

EPILOGUE

As I write this, my two children (his is a whole other story) are downstairs baking a cake; the superficially perfect family picture of normality; a reality that was painfully and painstakingly constructed, but one that I remain grateful for every day of my life. What I learnt during my infertile years, and what sufferers understand as obvious (versus what many doctors and non-sufferers ignore) is that infertility is not just a medical condition to be "treated" or "cured" with drugs and procedures. It is a crisis that profoundly affects virtually every aspect of a sufferer's life, to the extent that even when infertility treatments are offered with their hope of a resulting child, this psychological distress can be increased in ways that are rarely acknowledged or remedied. Whatever the outcome, this distress can continue for many years; and in cases of involuntary childlessness, potentially even forever.

I wrote the majority of songs in the four weeks leading up to my first IVF treatment. At that stage, we had been trying for a child for six years. I'd suffered 7 miscarriages. For the last two years I had failed to fall pregnant at all. Yet here I was, about to attempt one of the most emotional of medical interventions, and though there were theories, no-one had really found out why I miscarried. I was an internal mess of grief, confusion, inferiority and ferocity, continually asking "Why me?" whilst stripped of the everyday things I wanted to take for granted.

Songs was my cathartic outpouring, an unconscious art therapy in action, a way to cut through the fog of thoughts and loss of confidence. I believe it helped - not as a cure, but as a method to give voice to the turmoil and make it visible; it allowed me to stand outside the circle and name the pain.

'Songs' then remained in a drawer for over a decade, till Dr Susan Bewley, my consultant at the high risk pregnancy unit got in touch again during the pandemic lockdown; I'd given her an early copy during discussions over my second pregnancy to explain my need for a c-section; Dr Bewley is a strong advocate of natural birth, but I'd hoped the poems would demonstrate the reasons (my infertility history coupled with a difficult birth with Bella) for my lack of trust in my own capabilities and my phobia of things going wrong; I wanted to hand over responsibility to the doctors and let them effectively take me out of the equation. She not only agreed to the c-section, but took a genuine interest in the poems, even using two in the front piece of her book. It was her nudge during lockdown that opened the drawer, and it has been with her help, editing and mentoring, that this book has been published. We both agree, despite the passing of time, the words and themes are as relevant today as they were when they were first written, if not more so:

Infertility has always been with us, but it is a spreading disease; birth rates are falling, potential parents, for whatever reasons, are starting their families later, some even say chemicals and our modern lifestyles are a factor. One couple in seven will fight infertility and one in four pregnancies ends in miscarriage, so even if infertility isn't affecting you directly, it is undoubtedly having an impact on someone close to you.

Understanding infertility is multi layered and complex, especially when the postcode lottery, the high cost of treatments and limited window of time are considered. Add to this the variety of childbearing losses from never falling pregnant to ectopic pregnancies, miscarriage and stillbirth, and a truth emerges that illustrates every situation is different and unique in its own right. But whilst emotions can't be measured and pain can't be quantified, all these events are linked together by one thing all sufferers understand: grief.

I offer songs not as a story of success, but as an expression of suffering, trauma and the rollercoaster ride of infertility in the hope it may shine a light on the shared, often silent emotions of infertility and be a vehicle of connection for anyone who feels isolated and alone. In these pages, I hope you are recognised.

I still believe that it is this element, the emotional, because it can't be seen or proved, that isn't given enough currency regarding infertility. And yet I think it holds a golden key, not necessarily for success, but certainly for individual understanding and as a route to greater peace.   It is my hope that through this recognition of emotions, 'Songs' will put a spotlight on the potential that art holds as a healing force; I believe we ignore this bridge at our emotional peril.

Kate x

For further information, help and resources please head to
www.songsformyunbornchildren.com

THANK YOU

For help and encouragement: My lovely John, Ella, Nicola and Sue.

For the beautiful photo of Charlie used on the front cover, thank you to Alexandra Joseph of Alexandra Joseph Photography. You take the best.

This volume would not have been published without the help of Dr Susan Bewley. A huge debt of thanks is owed to her.

She not only guided in the births of both my children, but also in the creation of this book, reading, mentoring, supporting and advising.

In all my experiences with doctors, she was the one who took the time to listen.

Thank you xxx

Printed in Poland
by Amazon Fulfillment
Poland Sp. z o.o., Wrocław

62256157R00081